CONSENSUAL
SUICIDE

Published by Mindstir Media, LLC

45 Lafayette Rd | Suite 181| North Hampton, NH 03862 | USA

1.800.767.0531 | www.mindstirmedia.com

Printed in the United States of America

ISBN-13: 978-1-7355880-1-8

CONSENSUAL SUICIDE

PART ONE

AUGUSTINE ROGERS

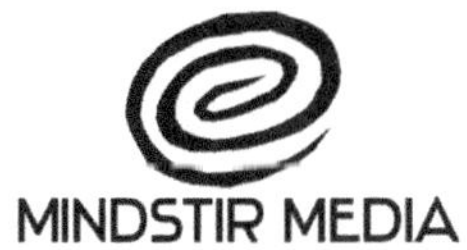

MINDSTIR MEDIA

TABLE OF CONTENTS

PREFACE

I MUST GIVE CREDIT FOR THIS BOOK TO MY MOTHER, who is a retired nurse. She is still alive, but she has fought many medical battles that have prevented her from living a full life. One of those battles was breast cancer, which was detected in, first, one breast and, then, the other. These diagnoses were discovered eighteen years apart.

My mother was a registered Dietition years before she became a practical nurse. Despite of moms remarkable credentials, she prepared and served her family harmful foods, unknowingly. She used to ask me what I wanted to be when I grew up, and I always said, "A nurse, just like you! The idea of becoming a dietitian wasn't even in the back of my thoughts. Little did I know that many decades later I would have a profound interest in health and ones well being.

I grew up eating pork, beef, chicken, turkey, fish, and some wild game, just like many others who were raised in the South. These meats were the main staples in our community and most of the world. The five basic food groups and the food pyramid, which are 2 proteins, 3 milk and dairy products, 4 fruits and vegetables, and 5 fats and sugars. Children and adults have no Idea that certain foods play such an important role in our over all health.

As the years progressed, I watched as my close relatives, like my beloved grandmother and grandfather, died. My mother's sister had her leg amputated from the hip. Their brother died. All of this death was caused by the big C — cancer. Everyone ate the same (some more than others), and some ate more exotic foods because of their affluence, yet none were able to put the puzzle pieces together in order realize how systematic consensual suicide had invaded their lives.

This was when I realized that something was very wrong with medicine. Even though my mother was a nurse, and her sister was married to a doctor, they were not immune to severe illnesses. I wondered, How did these severe illnesses and deaths happen? And more importantly, why didn't they know how to prevent them from happening? Why didn't their physicians look outside the box and take the necessary steps to stop the progression of their cancers and prevent them from returning?

I had a lot of questions, but there were no answers to be found. After watching my mother's health challenges, I knew, deep down in my being, I had to be the catalyst for change going forward.

I believe doctors should educate patients about the need for lifestyle changes and what necessary nutrients are needed for our bodies to remain in balance. Doctors should cease and dissist their positions of being drug dealers and pushers. It's time to have real patient/doctor conversations that are not one sided.

When I started my family, I, too, got caught up in the rat race of balancing work and family life. Short cuts were taken to make life easier and run smoothly throughout the day. We introduced the microwave into our home because we believed it would make life easier. We began to purchase quick "foods" to prepare for our beloved families, that would fit the hectic schedules loaded with activities that took us away from each other, rather than bring us closer.

We had no idea the damage we were inflicting on our children and significant others. Because of the way we were raised, the statement "I am grown and can eat whatever I want" was put into play. Well, that is true, but there are consequences that we will have face later on down the road because of our present-day decisions.

THE BEGINNING OF CONSENSUAL SUICIDE:

HOW DID I GET HERE?

I MENTIONED THE DIETS that most of us born in the South consumed that consisted of pork, beef, chicken, turkey, fish, and some wild game. These meats were cooked in lard, for the most part, or smoked. Desserts, which consisted of massive amounts of sugar and lard for the crust of pies, was a mainstay in our home when I was growing up. Fatback or ham hocks were used in greens, and real butter was used in macaroni and cheese. This type of diet has little to no nutritional value because of the way it is prepared. With this type of toxic food consumption comes visits to the doctor.

"Why?" you ask.

"Because of the artery clogging meats and unhealthy fats we say we love and can't do without. Because of the excessive weight gain, which has become uncontrollable. Because of the inability to walk a flight of stairs without being completely winded," I say.

We make statements such as "My mother cooked this way and lived to be ninety; therefore, so can I." This is where being an advocate for your health takes presidence over such statements. Here are some real facts about the consumption of meats and unhealthy fats. It's worth taking a closer look:

It's said that one man's meat is another's poison, but these days, it seems, increasingly, that every man's meat is every man's poison. Research published in The British Medical Journal; National Cancer Institute in Maryland; Department of Epidemiology and Biostatistics; Cambridge University Press PDF suggests eating processed meats including red meat, greatly increases one's risk of dying from heart disease or cancer. So do you think this is a major concern or a scare tactic?

In 2012, a study was published in the Archives of Internal Medicine, Harvard School of Public Health Harvard Medical School Boston, MA; which tracked about 121,000 participants for approximately twenty-eight years. What they found was that red meat consumption was associated with the overall increased risk of mortality, including cancer and cardiovascular diseases.

EXCERPTS FROM THE WORLD HEALTH ORGANIZATION

The World Health Organization (WHO), published an article in Issue 27 summer/Fall Cancer prevention Article - NY Presbyterian Cancer Care; and The American Cancer Society in Oct. 26, 2015 with claims that processed meat causes cancer. Some may think it's cool to consume 50 grams of processed meat daily (the equivalent of about two slices of lunch meat), but this study found that this amount of meat can increase the risk of cancer in humans by 18 percent. I would be remiss if I did not to mention that processed meat has officially been classified by the American Cancer Society as "carcinogenic to humans," and unprocessed red meat more than likely is as well. Evidently, while it is still said that red meat has some nutritional value, consuming large quantities of meat isn't good for our health.

Let's break it all down. Eating red meat isn't good for you, and you have an ironclad guarantee from the cattle. Leave it in the pasture and live better lives. Eating excessive amounts of red meat has been linked to a plethora of health problems, from an increased risk of colorectal cancer, hormone-sensitive breast cancer, diabetes, and Alzheimer's disease to mental health issues such as depression. It may not hurt to mention the fact that the strongest animals in the world are not carnivores, but herbivores.

As the evidence suggests that eating meats causes disease (dis-ease) in the body, the question is, What do I do now? Well, what the medical industry hopes is that you immediately seek medical attention from a professional licensed to "practice medicine." Before we go any further, let me expose the "doctor" also known as the "physician."

PHYSICIAN

First, let's expose the so-called father of medicine, Hippocrates. The next few pages will expose the lies that have been told and that have played out for centuries. They continue until this day. The truth will set you free, if your mind is open to receive it.

EGYPT: ANCIENT EGYPTIAN MEDICINE

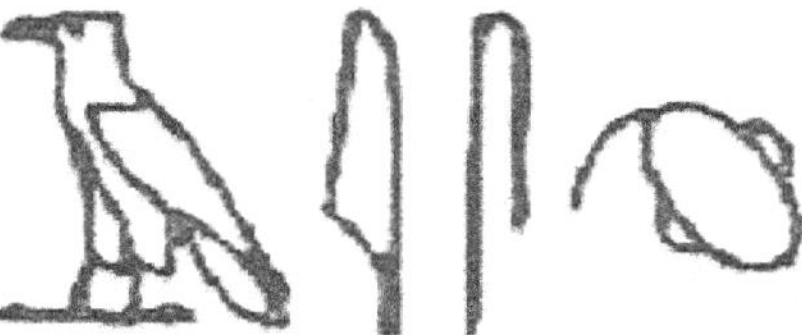

The *Edwin Smith papyrus,* written in the seventeenth century BC, contains the earliest recorded reference to the brain. Ancient Egypt developed a large, varied, and fruitful medical tradition. Herodotus described the

Egyptians as "the healthiest of all men, next to the Libyans" because of the dry climate and the notable public health system they possessed. According to Herodotus, "the practice of medicine is so specialized among them that each physician is a healer of one disease and no more." Although Egyptian medicine, to a considerable extent, dealt with the supernatural, it eventually developed a practical use in the fields of anatomy, public health, and clinical diagnostics.

Medical information in the Edwin Smith papyrus may date to a time as early as 3000 BC. Imhotep, in the third dynasty, is sometimes credited with being the founder of Ancient Egyptian medicine and with being the original author of the Edwin Smith papyrus, detailing cures, ailments and anatomical observations.

The Edwin Smith papyrus is regarded as a copy of several earlier works and was written c. 1600 BC. It is an ancient textbook on surgery that is almost completely devoid of magical thinking and describes in exquisite detail the examination, diagnosis, treatment, and prognosis of numerous ailments.

Hippocrates is considered the father of medicine, enemy of superstition, pioneer of rationality, and fount of eternal wisdom. Statues and drawings show him with a furrowed brow, thinking hard about how to heal his patients.

And today, the internet is full of claims that, if you follow a supposedly Hippocratic diet of raw organic foods or concentrate on one of his alleged favorite foods, such as watercress, you will be healed.

The most famous of the treatises linked to his name over time is the Hippocratic Oath which has sometimes been taken by medics as they vow to uphold ethical standards in their profession. And what a model it offers. In the oath, doctors are to keep away from abortion and euthanasia. They must not blurt out their patients' secrets, and they should not have sex with their patients — man or woman, free or slave.

Interestingly, the Hippocratic Oath has nothing to do with Hippocrates. So why has it been attached to his name?

THE REAL HIPPOCRATES

The reality is that, not just the oath, but the sixty or so other ancient Greek treatises on medicine that we call the Hippocratic Corpus, are all anonymous. They were written over many centuries in different Greek dialects. They also have different ideas about the body and healing. Today, classics scholars are clear that they can't all have been written by one man.

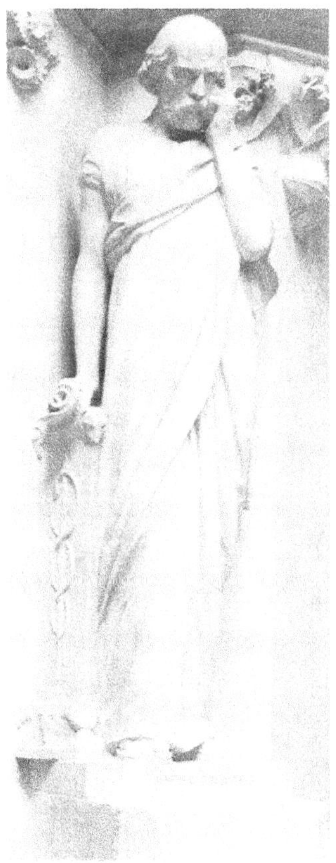

Hippocrates thinking hard at the Natural History Museum in Oxford.
pauJLeu, cc BY-NC

The philosopher Plato gave the only near-contemporary account of the real Hippocrates behind the myths. Hippocrates was known well enough as a physician in the ancient world that people would recognize him by name. From Plato, we learned that Hippocrates came from the island of Cos, close to the coast of what is now Turkey and taught medicine for a fee. He was an Asclepiad, which could mean one of a family claiming descent from the god of medicine, Asclepios, or just a healer. But it is not clear what beliefs he held about healing.

Anything else you read about the historical Hippocrates is made up. There are no recorded dates about his existence. Plato's references would put him at around 430 BC, but if you read any firm birth and death dates, they are figments of someone's imagination.

Making Up a Story

Hippocrates is an extreme example of our human desire to tell a story and to establish founders. Different facets of the surviving medical treatises from ancient Greece were taken out and merged to create his personality and, later, a whole biography. People made up family trees for him and speculated, with no evidence, on his education and character.

So we've imagined Hippocrates as a caring and attentive person simply because some ancient Greek treatises talk about how he observed patients very carefully. Because the treatise *On the Sacred Disease* talks about seizures as coming, not from the gods, but from an imbalance of phlegm in the body. We think of Hippocrates as someone who rejected anything superstitious. And because one surviving treatise is the Oath, Hippocrates is also linked to high moral standards.

What Does the Oath Really Say?

Most of the lines in the Oath are not about treating patients at all. Instead, they are about physicians teaching each other's sons without charge and taking care of their old teachers.

Whichever group of ancient physicians came up with this document, their first concern was with their identity as a group. Even the famous lines about euthanasia and abortion are far less straight forward than we expect. There is no ban in the Oath on euthanasia (as interpreted using our modern definition) as an option to end the suffering of a person who is battling an incurable condition. Kalo thanato is Greek, meaning "good death," but for an ancient Greek, a good death was that of a young man in his prime dying on the battlefield. Instead, the Oath suggests a much broader concern for keeping control of potentially fatal drugs, rather than handing them out to those who could misuse them.

As for abortion, the Oath says: "I will not give an abortive pessary." One of the most common infinitives (to give) is used here which means it is hard to know whether the sense is just "to hand over" or a more technical "to administer." And it leaves open the possibility for an abortive drug to be taken by another route — by mouth — as administered by a physician. Maybe the real worry in the Oath here is about the pessary as a particularly potent mode of administration, or again about letting drugs taken from the hands of a physician be given to those who might misuse them.

And as for the "no sex with patients of either sex" clause, this raises the possibility that the Oath was not a normal part of ancient medicine, but rather a very special document put together in some unusual local situation. Perhaps physicians had been doing precisely this, and the patients had completely lost faith in those who claimed that they could heal them.

Linking all these very different ancient Greek documents together and tying them to the name of Hippocrates became common practice just a few centuries after he lived. Perhaps it makes us feel better to see one, humane person rather than a faceless committee at the origins of medicine and medical ethics. And not just any person, but this idealized figure, the perfect physician who is more knowledgeable and more caring than any living physician we are likely to ever meet.

Throughout the history of medicine, we have made up the character of Hippocrates to fit what we think physicians, or medicine itself, should be like. Even the Oath has been edited to fit different societies.

But isn't it time to talk about medicine without always nodding to a shadowy figure from the past?

CONSENSUAL SUICIDE:

THE DOCTOR!

AFTER HEAVY CONSUMPTION of an unhealthy lifestyle, what transpires next is sickness and dis-ease. These words ring loudly to the ears of the plethora of physician$ and the pharmaceutical industry. Pawns in the game of living we are, and we accept our positions willingly, freely, and ignorantly. After our weight and vitals are taken, in comes the predator, the doctor, and we begin to recite the list of symptoms we've been experiencing. He or she is writing or typing as we speak, and sometimes not even lifting an eye to listen to our complaints. This is spoken from experience.

Next, he/she listens to our lungs, heart, checks our reflexes, looks in our ears, and checks our eyes and throat. He/she then proceeds to pull out his/her prescription pad and writes several prescriptions that he/she has very limited knowledge about. Sometimes, we, the patients, are asked what we want him/her to prescribe. What the heck? He just booked his vacation, courtesy of the pharmaceutical representative that peddled these particular drugs at the expense of our lives. What do we do? What questions do we ask about the drugs prescribed? Do we just trust each word the doctor says without question, or do we get a second or third opinion? We don't complain. We just leave, get the prescription filled, pay the copay or the full price, take the drug, and complain to our friends, family, or anyone who will listen about the high cost of the medicine and about how something else hurts as a result of the synthetic drugs we know nothing about. We systematically consent to consensual suicide and are so programmed that we don't realize it.

There are a plethora of books on the market on the causes of cancer, how to prevent or reverse cancer, and what foods to eat to prevent cancer and other dis-eases. Some of us have several of them on our shelves at home and may have read them all, but never made a change in lifestyle. We watch the weight pile on five, ten, twenty pounds at a time. We look in the mirror one day and see our belly has laped over our pants/skirts; blocking the view of our feet. We see our clothes getting tighter and tighter, so we go to the store and purchase larger sizes. Because of denial, the sound of a tired sumo wrestler's breathing being hampered as he walks or climbs stairs becomes the norm for our breathing. We eat greasy foods, fatty foods, very little green leafy vegetables and fruits, yet we say we're healthy and will almost fight if you say otherwise.

Okay. Let's be straight forward. It wouldn't be a drug if it didn't come with that long list of, sometimes, deadly side effects. Here we go back to the doctor, and he prescribes another prescription to "help" with the side effects. WTH! I have another side effect from the first prescription for the side effects of that drug.

There's an overdue payment of apologies and call to action from physicans that must be paid to us, the abused patients, for this inadequate and disrespectful care. We must immediately rescind the consensual suicide agreements made written and verbally. We must not misrepresent ourselves as less than another based on financial status. We must not settle for what's thrown at us. We must take our power back!

THE PIS: PATIENT INFORMATION SHEET

Those in charge of writing the patient information sheet wrote confusing language, which is only understood by science majors or lawyers! So much trust has been placed in our physicians to the extent that we choose not to read the patient information sheet (PIS) provided by our pusher (pharmacist). If we took the time to read those PISs, we would throw those drugs away, or would we?

We have become an impatient people, in need of a quick pill fix, so we can go back to existing, not really living. This irresponsibility spills over into our entire existence. We are out of control robots, taking orders without asking any relevant questions, trusting all the wrong people and consenting to suicide consistently.

I'm not throwing stones here. My intent is to bring awareness to the deadly scheme the United States Department of Agriculture (USDA), Food and Drug Administration (FDA), American Medical Association (AMA), and American Heart Association (AHA) have in place. The list goes on for those who we rely on to keep us safe, but they are out to eliminate us systematically through tests, trials, selective and needless surgeries, as well as food recommendations proven to be carcinogenic.

Enough of my mind, let's look at some statistics from the Center for Disease Control (CDC) and WHO:

In 2017, the ten leading causes of death (heart disease, cancer, unintentional injuries, chronic lower respiratory disease, stroke, Alzheimer's disease, diabetes, influenza and pneumonia, kidney disease, and suicide) remained the same as in 2016. Causes of death are ranked according to the number of deaths. The following data was taken from the CDC's 2017 anual report (with added statements and comments by the author):

1. Heart disease. Number of deaths per year: 635,260.
2. Cancer. Number of deaths per year: 598,038.
3. Accidents (unintentional injuries). Number of deaths per year: 161,374.

4. Chronic lower respiratory diseases: 160,201
5. Stroke: 146,383
6. Alzheimer's disease: 121,404
7. Diabetes: 83,564
8. Influenza and pneumonia: 55,672

These are eye opening stats that should be looked at carefully and with concern. Do your own research and see that these totals continue to rise. Consentual Suicide is real and can be stopped by the one looking back at us in the mirror.

THE OVERWEIGHT AND OBESITY EPIDEMIC

16 February 2018
Key Facts:

- Worldwide obesity has nearly tripled since 1975.
- In 2016, more than 1.9 billion adults, eighteen years and older, were overweight. Of these, over 650 million were obese.
- Thirty-nine percent of adults, aged eighteen years and over (39 percent of men and 40 percent of women) were overweight in 2016, and 13 percent were obese.
- Most of the world's population live in countries where being overweight or obese kills more people than being underweight.
- Forty-one million children under the age of five were defined as being overweight or obese in 2016.
- Over 340 million children and adolescents aged 5-18 were over-weight or obese in 2016.
- Obesity is preventable.

WHAT DOES IT MEAN TO BE OVERWEIGHT OR OBESE?

The condition of being overweight or obese is defined as abnormal or excessive fat accumulation that may impair health. The body mass index (BMI) is a simple index of weight-for-height that is commonly used to classify whether adults are overweight or obese. It is defined as a person's weight in kilograms divided by the square of his height in meters (kg/m^2).

Adults

For adults, WHO defines being overweight or obese as follows:

- Someone who is overweight has a BMI greater than or equal to 25; and
- Someone who is obese has a BMI greater than or equal to 30.

BMI provides the most useful population-level measure of overweight and obese individuals as it is the same for both sexes and for all ages of adults. However, it should be considered a rough guide because it may not correspond to the same degree of fatness in different individuals.

Children Under 5 Years of Age

For children, age needs to be considered when defining if they are overweight or obese.

For children under 5 years of age:

- They are defined as "overweight" if their weight-for-height is greater than 2 standard deviations above the WHO Child Growth Standards median; and
- Obesity is a weight-for-height greater than 3 standard deviations above the WHO Child Growth Standards median.

Children Aged between 5-19 Years

The conditions of being overweight and obese are defined as follows for children aged between 5-19 years:

- Overweight is BMI-for-age greater than 1 standard deviation above the WHO Growth Reference median; and
- Obesity is greater than 2 standard deviations above the WHO Growth Reference median.

FACTS ABOUT THE OVERWEIGHT AND OBESITY EPIDEMIC

Some recent WHO global estimates follow.

- Overall, about 13 percent of the world's adult population (11 percent of men and 15 percent of women) were obese in 2016.
- The worldwide prevalence of obesity nearly tripled from 1975 to 2016.
- In 2016, an estimated 41 million children under the age of five were overweight or obese. Once considered a high-income country problem, overweight or obese individuals are now on the rise in low- and middle-income countries, particularly in urban settings.
- In Africa, the number of overweight children under five has increased by nearly 50 percent since 2000.
- Nearly half of the children under five who were overweight or obese in 2016 lived in Asia.
- The prevalence of overweight and obese children and adolescents aged 5-19 has risen dramatically from just 4 percent in 1975 to just over 18 percent in 2016. The rise has occurred similarly among both boys and girls. In 2016, 18 percent of girls and 19 percent of boys were overweight.

- While just under 1 percent of children and adolescents aged 5-19 were obese in 1975, more than 124 million children and adolescents (6 percent of girls and 8 percent of boys) were obese in 2016.
- Being overweight or obese is linked to more deaths worldwide than being underweight.
- Globally, there are more people who are obese than underweight. The occurrence (more overweight/obese people than underweigh people) can be found in every region, except for parts of sub-Saharan Africa and Asia.

WHAT CAUSES SOMEONE TO BECOME OVERWEIGHT OR OBESE?

The fundamental reason someone becomes overweight or obese is because of an energy imbalance between calories consumed and calories expended. Globally, there has been:

- An increased intake of energy-dense foods that are high in fat.
- A decrease in physical activity due to the increasingly sedentary nature of many careers and professions, modernized modes of transportation, and increasing urbanization (microwave living). All forms of consensual suicide.

Changes in nutritional and physical activity patterns are often the result of environmental and societal associative changes encompassing development and lack of supportive policies in sectors such as health, agriculture, transport, urban planning, environment, food processing, distribution, marketing, and education. Below are some common health consequences of being overweight or obese:

- cardiovascular diseases (mainly heart disease and stroke), which were the leading causes of death in 2012;
- diabetes;

- musculoskeletal disorders (especially osteoarthritis, which is a highly disabling degenerative disease of the joints);
- some cancers (including endometrial, breast, ovarian, prostate, liver, gallbladder, kidney, and colon).

The risk for these noncommunicable diseases increases with increases in BMI.

Childhood corpulence (obesity) is associated with a higher chance of obesity and premature death and disability in adulthood. In addition to increased future risks, corpulent children experience breathing difficulties, increased risks of fractures, hypertension, early markers of cardiovascular disease, insulin resistance, and psychological effects.

The Double Burden of Disease

Many low- and middle-income countries are now facing a double burden of disease. While these countries continue to struggle with the issues of infectious diseases and nutritional famine, they are also experiencing a rapid upsurge in noncommunicable disease risk factors such as corpulence, particularly in urban settings. It is not uncommon to find nutritional famine and obesity coexisting within the same country, community, and the household.

Youth in low- and middle-income countries are far more vulnerable to substandard pre-natal, infant, and young child nutrition. Simultaneously, these children are exposed to excessive amounts of fat, sugar, salt, energy-dense (foods with high water content), and micronutrient-poor foods (foods our bodies need very small amounts of), which tends to be lower in cost but also lower in nutrient quality. These nutritional patterns, in conjunction with decreased levels of physical activity, result in skyrocketing increases in childhood obesity while nutritional famine issues remain unsolved.

Being overweight or corpulent, as well as their related noncommunicable diseases, are preventable. Supportive environments (households) and communities (open markets) are foundational in shaping people's choices, by making the choice of healthier foods (local farms/markets), regular physical activity (no gym needed) the easiest, no-excuse choice (one that is the most accessible, available, and affordable), and therefore, preventing the condition of being overweight or obese. At the individual level, people can:

- Avoid saturated fat and limit artificial sweeteners and high fructose.
- Focus on consuming nutrient-dense foods such as fruits, vegetables, legumes, whole grains, and nuts.
- Regularly engage in some form of physical activity (15-30 minutes of high intensity exercise or 60 minutes of moderate activity a day for children and 150 minutes spread through the week for adults, depending on level of fitness).

Individual responsibility can only come into full effect when people have access to a healthy lifestyle. Therefore, at the societal level, it is important to support individuals in following the recommendations above through sustained implementation of evidence-based and population-based policies that make regular physical activity and healthier nutrient choices available, affordable, and easily accessible to everyone, particularly to those who are less fortunate. An example of this is a policy which places a tax on sugar-sweetened beverages. The food industry could play a significant role in promoting healthy, nutrient-rich foods if what is in the best interest of the consumer were on their minds and hearts by:

- Limiting the amount of processing of "raw" foods;

- Ensuring that healthy and nutritious choices are available and affordable to all consumers;
- Ensuring the availability of healthy food choices and supporting regular physical activity practice in the workplace;
- Banning the marketing of foods high in sugars, salt and fats, especially those foods aimed at American children and teenagers of color.

These foods that cause sickness, dis-ease, and death are in our pantries and refrigerators and desk drawers at work right now!

GMO:

WHAT IS IT AND WHY IS IT BAD FOR YOU?

A GENETICALLY MODIFIED ORGANISM or GMO is a plant, animal, microorganism or other organism whose genetic makeup has been modified (changed from its original form) in a laboratory using genetic engineering or transgenic technology. This creates combinations of plant, animal, bacterial, and virus genes that do not occur in nature or through traditional crossbreeding methods. Genetic modification affects many of the products we consume daily. Following is a list of the most common genetically modified foods:

1. Corn
   Genetically modified corn turns up in many different products in the United States — and corn on the cob is the least of it. This crop is used to produce many different ingredients used in processed foods and drinks, including high-fructose corn syrup and corn starch. But the bulk of the GM corn grown around the world is used to feed livestock. Some is also converted into biofuels.

2. Soybeans
   The second largest U.S. crop after corn, GM soy is used primarily in animal feed and in soybean oil, which is widely used

for processed foods and in restaurant chains. In fact, soybean oil accounts for 61 percent of the vegetable oil consumed by Americans. It's also often used to make an emulsifier called soy lecithin, which is present in a lot of processed foods, including dark chocolate and candy.

3. Cotton
    Much of GM cotton is turned into cottonseed oil, which is used for frying in restaurants and in packaged foods like potato chips, oily spreads like margarine, and even things like cans of smoked oysters. Some parts of the plant are also used in animal feed, and what's left over can be used to create food fillers such as cellulose.

4. Potatoes
    A new kid on the block, this very recently approved GM crop is resistant to bruising and may produce less of a cancer-causing chemical, called acrylamide, when exposed to high heat. It has not yet seen adoption in the food supply but is expected to be.

5. Papaya
    Bred to withstand ringspot virus, which can destroy papaya plants, these genetically engineered "Rainbow" papayas were first commercially produced in the late 1990s. Much of the yield is grown in Hawaii.

6. Squash
    Zucchini and yellow summer squash have been commercially available in the United States since the mid- to late-nineties, though GM squash accounts for just 25,000 acres of farmland, by some estimates.

7. Canola
    GM canola is used to make oil for cooking, as well as margarine. It's also used to produce emulsifiers that are used in packaged

foods. By some estimates, 90 percent of canola grown in the United States and Canada is GM.

8. Alfalfa

   In a controversial decision in 2011, the FDA approved the commercial use of GM alfalfa that contains a gene making it resistant to herbicide. The crop is used mainly as hay for cattle.

9. Apples

   Another newly approved crop, this apple from a Canadian biotech company does not brown even after it's been sliced. It recently received FDA approval. The agency said it is safe to eat which means they may appear on supermarket shelves. I don't know about you, but I want to see the brown appear on my cut apple. There are other methods to keep the apple from turning brown as fast that are natural and perfectly safe for human consumption.

10. Sugar Beets

    More than half the granulated sugar in the United States comes from GM sugar beets, which have been in production since 2008. Though their use was temporarily halted due to safety concerns, production resumed in 2011.

Here is a list of the genetically modified foods we are already eating in the United States:

Corn	Cichorium Intybus	Rose
Canola	Rice	Apples
Alfalfa	Tobacco	Cotton
Potatoes	Sugar Beets	Beets
Rapeseed	Plums	Squash
Tomatoes	Papayas	Flax
Soybeans		

I believe this is a good point to end this section on genetically modified organisms. My intent, as always, is to convey my passion through words and actions, which hopefully are impactful enough to make a difference in just one life at a time and to leave a legacy for my children and grandchildren. If I am able to do these two things, then my mission is being accomplished.

PHYSICAL HEALTH/WELLNESS ELABORATED

WE DON'T GIVE THOUGHT TO THE SMALL, but necessary movements we make to do the simplest tasks every day. From turning on the stove to pushing a button on the microwave, energy is being expended to perform these tasks.

Hundreds of years ago, we would've had to go outdoors in the cold winter to chop wood for the wood-burning stove needed to keep the family warm through the night and into the morning. One can only imagine how much energy it took to complete this duty each day for weeks and months at a time. A vast amount of energy is used to keep the body warm during cold weather conditions, adding chores such as chopping wood uses more energy as well, yet it takes little to no energy to perform almost any other activity such as walking.. Today we have access to smart phones, notebooks and tablets, and laptops and computers to do what would've called upon a great amount of energy expenditure a few decades ago.

The result of today's automation and electronics has produced a busier and chronically sedentary lifestyle. However efficient it may be for tasks to be completed faster than before, for deadlines to be reached in rapid paces, there is a remote for every device in our lives, which causes us to use far less physical energy than our ancestors ever dreamed of.

A body in motion remains in motion. A body without physical activity is a body that settles and spreads. The muscles begin to atrophy, and after losing the strength to perform minute tasks, we become out of shape. The body becomes weak and loses the ability to perform basic physical tasks or engage in physical sports without an exhausting effort. Just when we think things couldn't get any worse, weakness comes in the sense of becoming more vulnerable to dis-ease and injury and difficulty recuperating from traumas. This is the lifestyle that has been consented to, the right to live a healthy lifestyle has been replaced with consensual suicide 100 percent. We want the right to do what we will with this vessel, but we don't want to accept the repercussions.

Exercise physiology studies how the body functions under physical exercise/activity. This physiology can determine the far-reaching limits of an individual's ordinary physical capacity to work. There are many stories of heroic proportions that I could mention, which are amazing and very true. What this says is that the human body can operate with far greater potential than we give it credit for, and there are many ways in which it can operate which are yet to be discovered.

Exercise is so important in the journey to live a healthier lifestyle. Performed correctly, exercise will strengthen the heart, lungs, bones, and, of course, muscles. Exercise also helps prevent illnesses, and it helps relieve depression and stress. Just exercising three to four times a week will benefit a healthier lifestyle.

Below is a Fitness Level test. It's not here just for your amusement either. Take the test to find out your level of fitness. Be truthful with yourself. There are no right or wrong answers. This is for you to self-evaluate, so, if necessary, you can make the necessary adjustments.

LEVEL OF FITNESS EVALUATION

Circle one response from column 1, 2, or 3 for each statement.

	1	2	3
1. I exercise daily.	Never	Sometimes	Always
2. I exercise, at least, 3-4x weekly.	Never	Sometimes	Always
3. I exercise, at least, 5-6x weekly.	Never	Sometimes	Always
4. I exercise less than 2x weekly.	Never	Sometimes	Always
5. I walk, run, swim, or engage in other forms of aerobic activity for, at least, 15 minutes each day.	Never	Sometimes	Always
6. I walk, run, swim, or engage in other forms of aerobic activity, at least, 45 minutes each day.	Never	Sometimes	Always
7. I enjoy using free weights.	Never	Sometimes	Always
8. I enjoy recreational exercise.	Never	Sometimes	Always
9. I enjoy biking.	Never	Sometimes	Always
10. I am consistent at exercising.	Never	Sometimes	Always
11. I make excuses not to exercise.	Never	Sometimes	Always
12. I watch my posture and correct it.	Never	Sometimes	Always
13. I pace myself in exercise so as not to overdo it.	Never	Sometimes	Always
14. I use hand weights and ankle weights for floor work.	Never	Sometimes	Always
15. I monitor my heart rate.	Never	Sometimes	Always
16. I gradually warm up before exercising.	Never	Sometimes	Always
17. I listen to my body and know when to rest.	Never	Sometimes	Always
18. When injured, I use rest, ice, elevation, and compression to care for my body.	Never	Sometimes	Always

19. I use proper form when using free weights.	Never	Sometimes	Always
20. I generally cool down following exercise.	Never	Sometimes	Always
21. I change my exercise routine.	Never	Sometimes	Always
22. I cross-train with aerobic activity, strength training, endurance, and flexibility.	Never	Sometimes	Always
23. I read articles on fitness tips and update myself on current information.	Never	Sometimes	Always
24. I walk, run, swim, or engage in other forms of aerobic activity, at least, 60 minutes each day.	Never	Sometimes	Always

SCORING: For every time you answered *never*, give yourself one 1 point. For every time you answered *sometimes*, this equals 2 points. For every time you answer *always*, this equals 3 points.

If you scored between 24 and 47, your level of fitness is described as leisurely, which means you probably aren't exercising enough to keep your body in top shape. If you scored between 48 and 64, you fall in the fit category. If you scored between 70 and 72, you are considered athletic. Keep it up!

EMOTIONAL WELLNESS AND HOW TO COPE

DID YOU KNOW THAT HOW YOU FEEL can affect your ability to carry out everyday activities, your job/business, your relationships, and your overall mental health? The way you react to your experiences and, sometimes, overwhelming feelings can change over time. Emotional wellness is your ability to successfully handle life's stressors and adapt to change and difficult situations. Something as simple as overstanding (understanding) that things don't happen to us physically and that it is the response to certain situations that we must come to terms with can make all the difference. What happens outside of us has no physical effect on us, but if we internalize each act, trauma, and situation, in turn, we'll get sick. Blood pressure rises, hearts palpitate, palms get sweaty, we get nauseous, etc.

Harmful Coping Strategies

In an effort to manage stress, we might have discovered one or more techniques for coping with stress that seem to work for a short period of time, but it turned out to be harmful over the long run. Following are some techniques that fall in one of two strategies:

Covering the symptom

- Distracting yourself from noticing stress symptoms
- Going out for happy hour after work for a few beers seems to be replaced by a false sense of ease and relaxation. This holds true for other forms of drugs as well, which helps an individual temporarily forget about what caused the stress in the beginning. Some people eat to cope with stress, while some shop.
- Dis-eases which come from the use of chemical abuse are esophagagial and stomach cancers. Other problems are ulcer disease and inflammation of the stomach and pancreas. In low doses, alcohol affects the liver's ability to produce sugar and, overtime, can cause alcoholic hepatitis and cirrhosis of the liver.
- Covering the symptoms is a strategy that conceals stress symptoms by reducing the body's sensitivity to them. When using alcohol to cope with stress, it induces a feeling of well-being. Alcohol is a depressant that relaxes the muscles and opens the blood vessels. This isn't a solution, but a temporary fix that will return as soon as its effects wear off. Compounding the problem, alcohol acts like a poison that kills the body's cells. There's a dulling of mental processes, perception, coordination, and motor functions. It later increases the risk of developing heart attacks and cancer and interferes with the immune system.

Beneficial Coping Strategies

There are two ways to deal productively with stress:

- Alter the sources of stress to reduce it
- Reduce your level of arousal

The single best stress manager is to use techniques that reduce the level of arousal that stressors can create. Remember that relaxation is like playing the piano — you can't simply decide to relax; you must train yourself to do it. Relaxation means the reduction of physiological arousal with actions such as abdominal breathing or systematic muscular relaxation.

Breathing: If you breathe irregularly, you disturb the gas exchange rate. This leads to a build up of the carbon dioxide levels in the body, which triggers a feeling of tightness in your chest and pressure in your body. Without a significant supply of oxygen to the body, waste products poison our bodies because they aren't properly removed. Your complexion may appear dark or blue because of a lack of oxygen in your blood. The digestion is also impaired. All body organs, muscles, and tissues become undernourished and may even deteriorate.

All this activity occurs in our bodies automatically, and we take it for granted. Our lives have become so busy that we don't take the time to stop and think, What is going on in my body? What is it doing with each breath that I take? We don't think about proper breathing techniques. Breathing exercises are effective ways of reducing:

- Stress
- Anxiety
- Depression
- Muscle Fatigue
- Irritability
- Tension

Breathing Abdominally (breathing with the diaphragm): This is the perfect form of breathing. For this technique to be beneficial, you should make it a regular program in your daily routine. As you practice holding your breath for a few seconds, you'll see how quickly the feelings of tension begin to develop in your chest and in other muscles of your body. On the other hand, an optimal pattern of breathing is breathing from the diaphragm. It reduces feelings of tightness in the chest, making it easier for the muscles to relax. Also, it slows the heart rate and reduces blood pressure.

Learning to Relax Your Muscles with Progression

There is a system that helps you become aware of major muscle groups and practice contracting and relaxing specific muscles. Over time, you will become increasingly sensitive to changes in muscle tension, and you will recognize when stress is coming on. Also, it will help muscles remain in a state of relaxation.

- Exercise specific groups of muscles to encourage relaxation.
- Your awareness increases how the muscles feel when they're relaxed.

When used together, both of the items above relax specific groups of muscles and induce a generalized state of relaxation.

Start with one muscle at a time and tighten it until you feel tension in the muscle. Once you are certain you feel tension, slowly relax the muscle. Pay close attention to how it feels as the tension is reduced. Create a system and work your way through all the groups of muscles in your body. Contract and release each muscle, at least, twice.

Relax first by lying flat on your back, with your eyes closed, and begin to breathe deeply. From distal to proximal, concentrate on your toes, allowing the tension to go from them. Systematically move up your body one muscle group at a time. Once you've reached your head, let all your cares, concerns, and pressures fall away. Maintain this relaxed state for ten minutes.

Practice this, at least, twice a day for thirty-sixty days; afterward, this practice will become a permanent part of your daily routine. You'll find you aren't able to function properly without it.

Roadblocks to Changes and the Answer to Overcome Them

Most of us have certain areas of our lives that could use a makeover; however, we make all sorts of excuses for putting off taking the necessary steps toward change. When ignored, these areas become problematic. There have been studies that have shown how an unhealthy lifestyle plays a major role in serious illnesses and dis-eases.

In this rat race of a world we live in, trying to build sustainable careers, start and raise a family, and stay ahead in the corporate world by competing constantly just to say, "I have it all," hundreds of millions of people neglect the importance of sustaining a healthy, balanced life, such as relaxing, eating nutrient rich foods for vital organs, and not taking life so seriously and, most importantly, overstanding oneself!

Instead, we live as if we'll have our youth forever because we bounce back after total exhaustion. But, one day, when it's least expected, that once young, agile warrior who lived in the fast lane begins to feel the result of a life of overindulgence and overwork. The panic only comes when the body begins to break down, then we realize we weren't as invincible as we thought! It's so unfortunate that, for most, this comes in the form of a heart attack or maybe a drunk-driving accident (DUI/DWI) or some other detrimental incident that causes pause, a pause long enough to step back and look at what has been created, left unattended with destructive behaviors.

Time and time again, I have made the statement that we house the power to change our own psychologies, our own minds. So many people put limits on their own abilities to become healthy/whole. Great emphasis has been self-placed on physicians. The ability to think for oneself has become obsolete. Becoming an advocate for one's own health is no longer a priority.

During the process of writing this book, I heard people from all walks of life create excuse after excuse for not taking the necessary time out to take care of themselves. When time is tallied up from the time of rising to the time of slumber, one would find a great amount of time for self-care. As one who is not close to being perfect, I find the time spent on social media (not guilty), reading emails throughout the day (guilty), wasted time on the phone, time watching the television (programs) adds up to time that could be spent on our bodies, our health, and our well-being. So, I ask, Who doesn't have time for life?

The psychology we tell ourselves is a false comfort and a psychological method to avoid accepting the challenge. "If I don't except the challenge, I won't fail." This is what we tell ourselves.

Social Barriers

We live in a heck of a society! The ideas of health in history show different periods had opposing thoughts than we do today. Years ago, smoking was fashionable. Today, it is a health hazard, and packages must contain that warning. We must watch what we eat and how we prepare foods. Heavy creams and butter aren't considered good for our health, yet at one time, they were.

I know I'm not the only one that remembers, long ago, the stereotype of the hoarse individual who was a chain smoker; now we look at the youthful and fit executive. This society of changing ideas poses a roadblock to changing successfully if individuals allow it with criticisms, paradoxes, and traditions.

Fear of the Unknown

We all have some form of fear in our lives. There are healthy fears and unhealthy fears. These are some of the questions that fear asks:

- What will it feel like to go through this change?
- How will I be different?
- Will the way I feel about my job, friends, or family change?
- Will my family, spouse, and friends have the same love for me?

These are real fears for so many people that hold them back from making the necessary lifestyle changes (i.e. career change, addressing issues within your relationships). I can attest to how childhood fears have held deep roots. There is a time when accidents, discipline, or unhappiness sets limits on imagination. The times that were set for play and fun in childhood are soon replaced with study and/or work. Some see growing up as a sad happening in life. Adults hold fears from their childhood, unknowingly placing limits on their greatest potential and achievements in life.

Along with fear of change comes rationalization. Rationalization is a process that negates any reason to change. Our human mind formulates what we use as excuses to resist any need to change. Here are a few...

- Denial
- Blame/Pointing the finger
- Procrastination/Fear of Loss
- And the biggie... Fear of Failure

How to Overcome Barriers

I, personally, am fond of the book *Who Moved My Cheese?* by Spencer Johnson. Here is a summary of the book. In this artful way, Spencer Johnson introduces the reader to his fable on how to cope positively with change. The story involves four characters who live in a maze: the mice, Scurry and Sniff, and two "little people", Hem and Haw. All is going well because they have found a huge source of their favorite food, cheese. Below are tips on how to identify the barriers preventing the change from being successful:

1. Write down only three attempts made toward change.
2. Write the reasons for the success or failure of these attempts.
3. Explore each reason deeply by gathering clues and start putting the puzzle together.
4. If you were successful, dig deeper and determine why. If you were unsuccessful, examine what may have helped to achieve the change.

This self-search approach will yield valuable keys for one to set out on a path toward a lifestyle change that will help you break out of that try-fail mental pattern by examining previously unsuccessful efforts. What this creates is a springbroad toward success. One of the best things you can do is form positive habits and change your habits and lifestyle to match your new goals.

Changing Habits and Lifestyles

Change should not be looked upon as a horrible time when we must be hard on ourselves. Three key elements make change successful, enjoyable, and positive. The elements that make change possible are awareness, support systems, and goal setting.

Awareness

Be informed and aware of how to manage stress. This is the first key element. We must become advocates for our own health. Try reading magazines for ideas or take fitness classes to learn about managing stress and how to develop an enjoyable lifestyle.

Support Systems

A crucial factor in a strong lifestyle change is a support system. Unsupportive friends and family pose insurmountable obstacles to individual success. Family, friends, and significant others should be very positive factors to this change. Support systems may not engage in the same activities but should always be there to congratulate and encourage us along the journey.

Goal Setting

Along with being aware and having a support system, another component toward success is goal setting. A process of setting visualized goals helps solidify the accomplishment of dreams and gives a larger road map to follow. Next step is to fill in the blanks of everyday living and decision making, such as what to eat and how and when to exercise and when to relax.

WELLNESS PLAN

Look at a wellness plan as a documented course of action that is geared toward achieving personal wellness. Personal wellness, then, implies a state of multidimensional health and complete satisfaction.

There are various dimensions to personal wellness, and each one must be nurtured, developed, and maintained for optimal overall well-being. Wellness is a state of mind. "We are what we become!" Wellness is an approach to health care that empowers and enables us to take charge of our own health and well-being. Utilizing a wellness plan provides us with the ability to live our best lives possible.

The beginning of the journey is knowing one's self. This is the fuel that will work in our lives. Once we begin to gain the knowledge needed, but more importantly understand, then we can work as a team to help with building skills, support, and the follow up that is needed to reach set goals.

There are six (6) foundational pillars that will be highlighted in this wellness plan, which are:

- Healthy Eating/Eating to Live vs. Living to Eat
- Physical Wellness
- Emotional Wellness
- Preventive Wellness
- Forming Positive Habits
- Surviving in an Unhealthy Workplace

The intention of this wellness plan is to bring awareness to what it means to be well, in every sense of the word. We will achieve this through knowledge garnered over a span of years of experience, education, and awareness of who I am.

The intent is to equip each one of us with an arsenal of wellness tools. These tools, when applied properly and consistently, will help us avoid the plethora of pitfalls constructed and set in motion by government and corporate entities to destroy life. We will show how it's strategically done, so through thorough preparation we can save the lives of our family and those we love.

Before embarking on any life change, the first thing to conquer, and by far the most difficult, is the mind-set. Our powerful minds were conditioned from conception. We were conditioned without question to believe certain rules and authorities. We were conditioned to love or not to love. We become very fond of things unknowingly, and we just like it! There are some foods that our mothers craved during pregnancy that reside within us; unfortunately, they seem to show up unsolicited.

The traits and characteristics of our fathers, even some of their appetites, manifest in us and our siblings. These are just a few demons we must take captive in our mind, if we choose to live a life of abundance, wellness, and wholeness.

Every page contained in this wellness/whole health plan comes by experience, hard work, and failure, which has been tried and tested. There isn't anything in here that I have not done myself and continue to do. Living is a daily task that should not be taken lightly. Being granted everyday mercies just to rise in the new day is a gift! What we do with that gift will shadow our entire lives, either in a healthy, productive way or in an unhealthy, unproductive way.

There is no way I could or would write this wellness/whole health plan without first going through the many pitfalls of living an unhealthy life. I read the books and articles the experts said we should read, and I

     CONSENSUAL SUICIDE

listened to the experts who I felt had the knowledge I needed to grow and become the best version of myself.

Even when I thought I was doing what was right, I found that I was still being deceived by those who I thought had my best interest at heart. Becoming an avid reader of everything pertaining to health was the spring board that launched me into action.

There were times that I took the advice of so-called professionals in the field of health. They all looked healthy, full of life, and enthusiastic about living well. The revelation was that so many "experts," for one reason or another, have chosen deception over transparency.

Transparency allows us to be human. Living in the shadows causes us to live outside of what we know is right. If we're not being transparent, we're living someone else's life. Remove the "F" from the word "life," and we have "lie." The whole truth about their struggles and what it took and takes to grow and succeed in life is what the world is looking for.

Healthy Eating/Eating to Live vs. Living to Eat

This is a huge topic and one that I tread on with caution. Food addiction, living to eat, and mindless eating are all connected. They all have one thing in common, which is an insatiable desire to consume foods that aren't healthy choices or proper portions. Usually these unhealthy foods are consumed during times when the body doesn't require fuel.

The focus is to bring clarity to the difference between eating to live vs. living to eat. It is vitally important to understand food and respect the purpose and need for life-sustaining, nutrient-dense food.

As I gather my thoughts and confidence to write about this topic, I'm reminded of the few times I sat watching a movie, and during the commercial break, they flashed those tasty, yet addicting Doritos ads. I've had an addiction to Doritos for some time now and still must talk my mind down when passing them at the checkout lane. I know all about food cravings, comfort foods, and other favorite foods we grew up eating that have been staples in our pantries since we left our parents' homes. We ate most of what was placed before us with no thought as to whether it was good for us or not then. As adults, that mentality grew with us; therefore, we think those same foods are good for us now.

Time keeps moving, even when we're standing or sitting still; therefore, let's start where we stand by taking control of what we eat. It is important that you become an informed shopper, someone who knows what foods are needed to sustain life and which are GMOs that were created to be sustainable over an extremely long period of time, which have side effects that will kill every organ in our living bodies.

First, allow me to explain what a GMO is. "Genetically Modified Organism" is what the acronym stands for. How do they do it you ask? Well, they, scientists, create DNA to synthesize compounds artificially, rather than extracting these compounds from natural sources.

Did you know that genes can be deleted, turned on and off, or new ones can be created by DNA sequences on a computer? These sequences do not occur in nature. This is a statement from consumers and the U.S. Patent Office.

The saying "the devil is in the details" is a true statement. Companies don't want unsuspecting consumers to know where or how the foods they consume and feed to their families comes from. Why? Profit! Greed!

Genetically engineered fish and animals — dehorned cattle, naturally castrated pigs, chicken eggs that contain a pharmaceutical agent — are all in the genetic experimentation pipeline. This is what they are working on now. Some of which are being sold now.

Again, this is consensual suicide when we allow them to control what we consume without reading, investigating, researching, and becoming our own health and wellness advocates.

Here we go. Fish are being sold in Canada; the whereabouts are being withheld. The only hold up from the United States taking part in these sales is due to "labeling complications."

A 2013 *New York Times* poll states that 75 percent of respondents said they would not eat GMO fish. Two-thirds said they would not eat meat that was a GMO. Check out apples the next time you purchase them. Do they turn brown once bitten or cut? If they don't, beware. That's a GMO apple.

RNAI: is a gene portal protein which turns genes on and off to create specific traits. An apple called the Nonbrowning Artic apple was engineered with RNAI to turn down the brown or mushy expression gene.

We've become oblivious to the Nonbrowning apples, the seedless tomatoes, the seedless cucumbers, and so on and so forth. Consumer beware.

We consent to consensual suicide every day we live and breathe. Time to wake up and not smell the coffee. It's time to see the deception and act accordingly. We need not be ashamed to ask our bodies how they feel after that meal or snack. How is our attitude being portrayed by others throughout the day? Do we feel sluggish, fatigued, or agitated?

Are there or have there been episodes of frequent headaches, migraines, or body aches that are not from exercise, sinus infections, joint aches, and/or unexplainable pains that we blame on age?

In my opinion, it is so important that it should've been a prerequisite before graduating from high school, and that is to learn to listen to the messages our bodies give every day, messages pertaining to the innermost parts that sustain our lives. Those messages that we dismiss deliberately. I know that I'm not the only one that has experienced this; otherwise, this wellness plan would not exist.

Here's the real deal. Our parents did what they had to do to keep us alive. They put on the table what they thought was good nutrition. We cannot blame them for their lack of knowledge about food.

For those of you who are like me, we knew that our parents struggled to put food on the table, and the last thing we thought about was whether the food we were eating was good or bad for us. No thought was given to it whatsoever.

Now it's our time to ensure that what we purchase, cook, and serve to our families is quality food, food that isn 't genetically modified. We must be proactive and become advocates for our own health and well-being.

Understand that only you care about your family. Understand that the FDA, AMA, CDC, and every other organization governs how food is grown, whether farmers are using the fertilizers that they instruct them to use on crops or not.

We are what we eat, and we are also what we don't eliminate. If we continue to eat "dead foods," there is no way our organs, whose function is to keep and maintain our bodies in homeostasis (balance) would have the ability to function properly.

It's like drinking a glass of formaldehyde and expecting life to continue with no interruptions. That's ludicrous! Don't take my word for it. Go to YouTube and watch *What the Health* and every other documentary pertaining to what "they" (the governmental-corporate packs) allow in the foods we eat daily.

We must be mindful that these tactics have been carefully studied by marketers. These ads are designed to work on our salivary glands, our desire for quick energy, or so-called quick food. Look at this as a trick to take our attention away from what is important at that moment. We aren't hungry. These commercials/ads are geared to work on our senses. What must be adjusted are our thoughts and ideas revolving around hunger and taught behaviors.

HUNGRY?

WHAT IS IT AND HOW DO I KNOW WHEN I AM REALLY HUNGRY?

How can we define hunger? So many people, myself included, had the idea that hunger was when our stomaches growled, we got a slight headache that got worse the longer we waited to eat, or we became weak, felt faint, and sometimes began to shake a bit. Well, let me be the bearer of bad news to the masses. All those symptoms are just the opposite of being hungry. They are all derived from external stimuli from the unhealthy foods that we've consumed. They are showing up in familiar ways, bidding us to provide more of the unhealthy foods/snacks we've become accustomed to. Toxins are released through many mediums in our bodies that we count as negative sensations in our bodies.

Hunger begins in the mouth and ends in the throat. I must note that the true signs of hunger are subtle. When we get hungry, our mouths begin to salivate and we feel and hear that all to familiar belly growl. This is when we get in trouble with unhealthy foods/snacks.

Once we begin to eat properly, our bodies react to hunger differently than before. We become aware of our bodies' systems and functions.

True hunger is when our mouths begin to salivate, then our throats feel the sensation of hunger. That's when we need to eat!

Preparing Healthy Foods

Healthy eating isn't just preparing a meal and placing it before our families. Healthy eating entails gathering, cleaning, and preparing of "live food." There is energy in the process that will never be experienced with processed foods (dead, no form of life).

There is something to be said for family unity, when everyone shares in the preparation of meals. This is a lost treasure. In turn, we've exchanged eating to live for living to eat. The poisons served at breakfast, lunch, dinner, and the snacks we eat in between should cause an anger to rise from deep within. Unfortunately, the anger would be misdirected. Instead of being angry at those who created and marketed these products, the focus and the blame rests upon those of us who purchased, cleaned, prepared, and served these poisons to our families. We gave up our human right to be informed, educated, and knowledgeable. Wisdom is only seen as the owl sitting atop a tree or pole. We've thrown away our birthright. We didn't get a dime for it! In return, we have been and are given death on a gold plate.

Reading is fundamental, people! We should be reading about everything we intend to feed our families and ourselves. When I began my journey toward living my best life, my family thought I'd lost my mind. When I went to the market to purchase food for my family, I literally spent two to three hours in the market, just reading labels. There was no way I was going to be responsible for feeding death to my family whom I love dearly.

Knowledge is power! If you can't pronounce it without breaking it down phonically, do not buy it, let alone consume it or use it in any way. Whatever it is, it doesn't belong in or on a living body.

We need to take time and read what we put in our baskets before we do. It's time out for just buying what we can "afford." When will we begin to purchase what will sustain our lives and the lives of our children and grandchildren? Or do we really care? When we know better, I hope we'll do better.

I am fully aware that most Americans do not get the required amounts of servings of fruits and vegetables in their daily intake; it's obvious by my last statement. Fruit roll-ups (sugar), fruit cups (sugar), so-called fruit smoothies sold at the markets and health food stores (labeled as natural, but sugar is disguised by other names), and so-called health drinks do not fall under the category of live foods.

We are a society of gluttons. Yes, I said it. Gluttons! We eat on the run and make excuses for why we can't prepare a decent breakfast before going to work. Oh! Don't even mention preparing a hot breakfast for our children before we send them off to school, summer camp, or any other organized sport/activity. Instead, they're fed glue-based treats disguised as pastries, with fake strawberries or other eye-appealing artificial ingredients engineered to prey upon them.

On our lunch breaks, we run like crows to road kill to our favorite bodega or other takeout establishment, only to gorge ourselves on the quickest widow-making burger or plate of cholesterol-laden fries from McDeath (McDonald's) or BugerKill (Burger King). Are you awake yet, or should I continue? No! Okay, here's more to masticate on.

Moreover, this microwave, take-out society that we've been programmed into has created a society of mindless robots. We've been electronically lobotomized willingly, but unknowingly by others' intentions. We no longer can think for ourselves, choose for ourselves, or decide for ourselves.

Everything is streamed into our sub-consciousness willingly yet unknowingly. We've chosen to stay connected with the majority, instead of choosing to disconnect with the minority. Don't believe the hype that there's strength in numbers; that's not always the case. This is where discernment is needed.

We only get one life, and what we do with that one life is purely our choice, not the masses. We do, however, need someone, at times and only for a season, to give us the push, to give us the motivation to get started.

Whose life is this we're living? Is it ours to do with what we please? To live haphazardly, minds decaying because of the lack of desired knowledge and dissociative behaviors that weren't even heard of over 65-70 years ago? Really! Is this what we think, what we believe? Or are we to care for this one life we've been given, as if it were the only one we will ever have in this lifetime? The choice is ours to make!

Beginning a healthy eating regimen takes dedication and a made-up mind to go all the way, no matter how difficult it may be or become. "We are what we eat" is a true statement that most take for granted. It is time to take back control of what we consume, especially for our children's sake. It is our responsibility to care for the bodies/vessels that house our spirits.

Physical Health/Wellness

This is a very touchy subject for most, especially women. I am a woman, of course, which gives me insight into our health, or the lack there of. I also believe in ancestral knowledge when referring to movement of the body and wellness.

If we traced our ancestral roots back, as some of us are doing today, we would see just how physical our ancestors were and had to be, in order to survive. They didn't have the luxury of purchasing a car that allowed them to travel for miles all around or drive to a grocery store to purchase items for their families.

Our ancestors toiled and labored in hot fields, tilling the hard and difficult earth to create rows that would be an incubator for precious seeds. By hand, with a bent over posture, walking in hot temperatures, this was done year after year. They watered, pulled weeds, and cultivated their crops. This was all very physical, hard labor that had to be done to feed their families. There was great pride in this accomplishment, and they gave praise and thanksgiving to their creator. Oh, what joy, when the seeds that they'd been nurturing became pods, sprouted, and became a flower that produced nutrient-rich food that was sustainable for life.

The process of tilling the soil took a great deal of sweat-producing energy as they worked long hours in the hot sun with no covering except for a hat or rag tied around their heads for protection against the hot sun. Our ancestral mothers drew water from a well to wash clothes on a washboard and for cooking and baths. This was no doubt strenuous work that had to be done. The convenience of turning on a faucet wasn't a thought. Everything done then took physical energy, thought (mental energy), concentration (mental energy), intention, purpose and, most importantly, love.

Physical wellness is swiftly becoming a relic today. Those who indulge in the plethora of physical activities are looked at as extremists, as over the top individuals. What's not being recognized is the fact that this is what we are supposed to be doing. Staying active from the cradle to the grave is what living is all about.

This idea about not wanting to be bulky and looking manly is preposterous and impossible without the use of steroids. Yes, the ability for a female who lifts substantial weights to gain muscle mass is obtainable. But the focus must be on bodybuilding. This is a very weak excuse for not wanting to do the work to obtain optimal wellness and whole health.

If you haven't recognized it yet, I am a straight shooter. Your time and life are precious, even though some may not see it as such. Life and time should be taken seriously, as they are synonymous with each other, especailly when it comes to how we care for the one and only body we have. This wellness/whole health plan is, as always, first to me, then to you, my readers.

Physical activity isn't a macho thing; women, especially, need to be active just as much or more than men. We are the ones who bare, nurture, and raise children. It really should be viewed as a requirement to be physical, for the sole purpose of being able to run behind them when they're small. Our children need us to be able to play with them in their younger years. Those who've had the honor of bearing or raising children know that those precious early years don't last long.

I am so blessed to have been able to raise five wonderful children, who I absolutely enjoyed having the pleasure of nurturing. We take life and living for granted far too much, never counting the cost of the damage we've done in the process.

Sometimes, it's a good idea just to visit nursing homes, retirement communities, and hospitals. Spend time with a few of the residents. Listen to their stories of old, when they had the use of their limbs. Some individuals are able, and some are unable to move about as they would like. The lives we have chosen to live will lead us in that direction prematurely, if these destructive behaviors that we have labeled as normal continue.

We are, emphatically, what we eat. Adding insult to injury, we are assuredly what we do not eliminate. Good, nutrient-rich food in, good food out; bad processed food in, bad food stays in, clogging our intestinal tract with toxins, fillers, and GMOs, preventing us from having a full elimination.

A regimen, minimally, of thirty minutes of vigorous exercise/ movement every day is all we need to live a well/whole life. There's a lot to say about walking ten thousand steps a day, according to the American Heart Association. American Heart Association's Recommendation for Overall Cardiovascular Health:

At least, thirty minutes of moderate-intensity aerobic activity, at least, five days per week for a total of 150 minutes or, at least, twenty-five minutes of vigorous aerobic activity, at least, three days per week for a total of seventy-five minutes or a combination of moderate- and vigorous-intensity aerobic activity.

And moderate- to high-intensity muscle-strengthening activity, at least, two days per week for additional health benefits. For lowering blood pressure and cholesterol average, forty minutes of moderate- to vigorous-intensity aerobic activity three or four times per week.

There are two (2) organs in each of our bodies which are incapable of exercise without our assistance. They are our heart and our lungs. Without the stimulation of activities such as walking, jogging, running, hiking, swimming, tennis or other strenuous activities that cause the heart rate to increase, these two organs would cease to function properly until they shut down completely. Weight bearing exercises build bone. Light weight lifting will promote bone growth, which is something we all need as we grow older.

In my next wellness plan, I will share more about how the body moves and exercises that facilitate muscle growth. First things first, though, this mind needs a lot of work before we begin to talk about putting together an exercise program.

Emotional Wellness

When I began writing this wellness/whole health plan, I realized this plan wasn't just for my audience. I realized it was, first, for me! My heart began to beat fast with each word I wrote, knowing that what I was about to share with the world was a real life, up close and personal version of me. I followed all the rules toward wellness and wholeness, except for one very important step, one that holds everything together when all about you is in chaos. You guessed it. Emotional Wellness!

Without sounding like a Dr. Phil or Oprah, I'll just share this — we are what we become. "What does that mean?" you ask. We envision ourselves as one thing or another throughout our lifetimes. We strategize, calculate, and create charts and vision boards as to what our lives should look like within a certain time frame. What we neglect to include are all the obstacles, mazes, towers, train wrecks, derailments, heartbreaks, setbacks, feelings of defeat, disappointments, failures, and the list goes on and on. How will we handle the inevitable life issues that will occur? Will we fold? Will we give up and give in? Will we throw away our dreams and give up on our goals or worse when circumstances arise? Our emotional wellness is just as beneficial as the other five, if we want to live the lives we were created to live.

We tend to internalize more than we should. If the question arose, do you know who you are? What would be the response, and would that response be accurate? It is good and healthy to study or get some insight about other faiths or religions. So much of how to control the mind from the Hindu monks is truly astonishing. What's more astonishing is that it took peering into the minds and thoughts of gurus to find that the power of the mind must be cultivated, trained. We have so many thoughts that pass through our consciousness during the twenty-four hours that are within a day. Let's just surmise that we all get about six to eight hours of sleep each night, which leaves us with about sixteen to eighteen hours to do all our daily tasks. The object that keeps us from successfully completing each task outlined for the day is concentration.

There are few that have conquered this thing called focus (concentration). Because of the world we live in with all the technology and gadgets, social media and programming, it's difficult, without practice, to master total concentration on one subject or task at a time. Thoughts flood our consciousness and subconsciousness, invading space that should be reserved for the task in front of us. Suddenly, a scenario from last night, last week, last month or even last year of unreconciled issues or projects comes to mind. Now we've forgotten what we were supposed to be focused on. Getting that focus back is difficult to master without, again, practice. Trust me when I say, I've been there and done that and am sure to revisit it again.

Concentrate: Focus on one thing, project, or task at a time. When another thought begins to surface, immediately make the shift to the

　　　CONSENSUAL SUICIDE

current task. This will have to be repeated several times. The key is to always draw focus back to the original thought. "Practice makes perfect practice."

Emotional baggage is another controllable focus thief. Every one of us has or is dealing with some sort of emotional baggage. The difference between those of us who've practiced and continue to practice letting go is we started the process. The first step is to recognize and say openly to ourselves, "It's not our fault." Even if fault lies with us, what's done is done. We must move on. "Easier said than done," you say.

Yes and no. We were all born with a choice. Choose life or choose death. Choose right or choose wrong. Choose to fight or choose to walk away. Choose to live a healthy lifestyle or die a miserable and unhealthy soul. We all have these choices!

Have you ever heard the phrase "Misery loves company"? Well, it's so true! Society and social media have shown us how to put our lives on display. The purpose is to garner attention and/or sympathy. The result is never good. Believe it or not, when we complain to people, have we ever thought that the recipient really doesn 't want to hear what we're complaining about?

We aren't looking for sound advice from that friend or associate. All we want to do is have them feel what we're feeling at that moment. It gives us some sick sense of relief only for a short season. Other emotional thieves that we invite into our spaces are gossip, being a busy body, degrading and putting down one another, ungratefulness, unkindness, greed, loftiness, and the list goes on.

I have a saying that I obviously didn't coin myself, but it says, "If whatever problem you're facing right now isn't able to be fixed by you, pray about it and leave it alone. If whatever problem you're facing right now is able to be solved by you, then do it without complaining. Everything isn't for us to control, fix, or sort out. The things that we can are clearly marked out, if we just stop, shut up and look."

Again, visit the nursing homes and have a conversation about life and the choices they've made. There is so much for us to be thankful for, yet we complain. Our emotional health and wellness are in jeopardy and has been for a long time.

Preventive Wellness

Preventive wellness, simply put, means measures set up to prevent diseases or illnesses from arising. Some of these measures include checkups, patient counseling, screenings and tests, and other means of acquiring necessary information in order to facilitate an accurate preventive plan, designed exclusively for that patient.

Taking the necessary steps to stave off unwanted illnesses and diseases is extremely important. Therefore, it is vital to have these screenings done early and on time. Life is but a vapor, here today and gone tomorrow. Let's make each day count!

Positive Habit Forming

It takes exactly twenty-one days to form a new belief. For us to believe, we must first commit to the fact that something is or isn 't! Is or isn't what? Good or bad, constructive or destructive, right or wrong?

When I decided to give up smoking cigarettes, I had gotten sick and tired of being sick and tired of smoking and having that smell on me and in my clothes and especially on my breath when I breathed or spoke. Cold turkey was how I did it; otherwise, it might not have been done at all. In addition, I made a list of all the things that could be accomplished without taking a smoke break. After making that list, I asked myself the following questions: What good benefits does smoking bring? Is this lifestyle getting me closer to my fitness goals, or is it holding me back, due to a lack of oxygen going into my blackened lungs?

Harsh, but so damn true! I smoked while in the military and hated every moment. Most soldiers do it to be in the "in" crowd and to look cool or grown. I really don't believe anyone begins smoking realizing the dangerous effects it has on our internal organs first, then appearing outwardly. Once hooked, it becomes difficult and sometimes impossible (so many think) to stop. Don't take it from me without seeing what the American Cancer Association has to say: About half of all Americans who keep smoking will die because of the habit. Each year, more than 480,000 people in the United States die from illnesses related to tobacco use. This means, each year, smoking causes about one out of five deaths in the United States. Smoking cigarettes kills more Americans than alcohol, car accidents, HIV/AIDS, guns, and illegal drugs combined. Cigarette smokers die younger than non-smokers. Smoking shortens male smokers' lives by about twelve years and female smokers' lives by about eleen years. Smoking not only causes cancer, but it can damage nearly every organ in the body, including the lungs, heart, blood vessels, reproductive organs, mouth, skin, eyes, and bones.

All right. After reading that, why would anyone choose to continue to kill themselves with deadly tobacco, all the while complaining about the nasty habit? I'll tell you why. Because it's an addiction. Making a conscious decision to form positive habits takes a made-up mind. Help is always here when needed. No one must do this alone, but the decision is a personal one.

Surviving in an Unhealthy Workplace

Finally, we will discuss the importance of working in a healthy work environment. It may seem as though this is an impossibility. How can one control what goes on in the workplace? Easy! It's time out for us to stop allowing our coworkers to dump all their junk on us. Stop allowing them to fill our heads with their garbage. We will tell our children what we want to hear and what we don't from them. Yet we sit back and take in everything thrown at us at our work place. Why?

Just like television, we become programmed to accept whatever is thrown our way gladly, not realizing the negative effects this behavior has upon us and our ability to function. Time is wasted at the dump, instead of on the work assigned. "No" is a beautiful word when used in the proper context. Learn to use it well. Is it necessary to develop a social network at work? No, but it can be a plus if joined with like-minded people.

In Conclusion

Use these tools in this wellness plan to your advantage. Fulfill all your goals. Make goals that are measurable because measurable goals allow us to see growth. They allow us to see whether we're on the right path or if we've ventured off a little. Measurable goals afford us the opportunity to regroup and get back on track. Everything outlined in this plan can be accomplished with intention. As mentioned in the beginning of this plan, I stated that this is the first of many wellness plans which describe the many aspects on total and optimal health and wellness for life.

Peace and Blessings,
Augustine Rogers, Health & Fitness Coach

ACKNOWLEDGE AND CREDITS

American Cancer Society

Ancient Egyptian Medicine

Archeives of Internal Medicine Harvard Health Publishing

British Medical Journal

Cambridge University Press

CDC (Centers For Disease Control)

Department of Neuroscience San Sebastian, Spain

Harvard Medical School

National Cancer Institute of Maryland

NY Presbyterian Cancer Care